MIND GAMES

MIND GAMES

Joan Leslie Woodruff

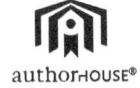
authorHOUSE®

AuthorHouse™
1663 Liberty Drive
Bloomington, IN 47403
www.authorhouse.com
Phone: 1-800-839-8640

© 2012 by Joan Leslie Woodruff. All rights reserved.

No part of this book may be reproduced, stored in a retrieval system, or transmitted by any means without the written permission of the author.

Published by AuthorHouse   10/15/2012

ISBN: 978-1-4772-8229-8 (sc)
ISBN: 978-1-4772-8230-4 (e)

Library of Congress Control Number: 2012919589

Any people depicted in stock imagery provided by Thinkstock are models, and such images are being used for illustrative purposes only.
Certain stock imagery © Thinkstock.

This book is printed on acid-free paper.

Because of the dynamic nature of the Internet, any web addresses or links contained in this book may have changed since publication and may no longer be valid. The views expressed in this work are solely those of the author and do not necessarily reflect the views of the publisher, and the publisher hereby disclaims any responsibility for them.

Contents

Day One	1
Day Two	3
Day Three	5
Day Four	7
Day Five	9
Day Six	11
Day Seven	13
Day Eight	15
Day Nine	17
Day Ten	19
Day Eleven	23
Day Twelve	25
Day Thirteen	27
Day Fourteen	29
Day Fifteen	31
Day Sixteen	33
Day Seventeen	35
Day Eighteen	37
Day Nineteen	39
Day Twenty	43
Day Twenty-One	45
Day Twenty-Two	49
Day Twenty-Three	53
Day Twenty-Four	55

Day Twenty-Five 57
Day Twenty-Six 59
Day Twenty-Seven 61
Day Twenty-Eight 63

My Other Books 69

You are never going to be perfect.
I am never going to be perfect.
Perfection is not attainable.
Happiness is always transient.
Makes you want to give up already.

Then, as if life isn't difficult enough, neuroscience reveals our brains are wired from birth toward negative thinking. Negative thinking helps us expect and see danger because we know it's out there, which aids our survival. Unfortunately, negative thinking also makes us miserable; but, we do it so often, we are experts in manufacturing our self created misery.

You know this: If you do something often enough, you're going to get really, really good at it. No wonder we are experts when it comes to seeing "the glass is only half full." Our negative circuits are always busy!

Why try, right?

The answer is, you should try. Life is short. While you are here, you want to enjoy as much of your life as you can. (Note: ***If you are depressed, see your doctor, this isn't for you!***)

While a young therapist, I noticed my patients were much happier when they **perceived** their day's chores positively. I came up with a check list which asked them to rate the activities of their days, keeping track for several weeks. The actual chore/activity/work had little to do with happiness. It was their **perception** of it that mattered. The American Occupational Therapy Association (AOTA) invited me to present the results of this research at an annual AOTA convention in Anaheim, California. Afterward, because I didn't know what else to do with the results, I donated my research to the National Institute for Mental Health (NIMH). I have no idea if they looked at it. I do believe it strongly supported that thoughts lead to mental health **quality**.

During postgraduate work I studied many theorists, who I began to think of as theory couriers. Their fields included psychoanalysis, Adlerian theory, existentialism, person centered therapy, Gestalt, behavior therapy, cognitive behavior therapy, reality therapy, feminist therapy, postmodern approach, family system therapy, integrative therapy, and many more. Those whose work transferred more into measurable science than theory are the ones whose work you will recognize in various flavors throughout this workbook. They are: AAron Beck, MD; Jon Kabat-Zinn, PhD; Byron Katie; James W. Pennebaker, PhD; Dan Siegel, MD; Daniel Amen, MD; James Gordon, MD; Thich Nhat Hahn; and my favorite, Socrates.

I write this active participation **workbook** just for you. Think of this collection of exercises as something created specifically for your benefit. If you take a sincere and active part in this workbook, and you truly work all the exercises, by the time you are finished, you will be living your life more fully. This is not therapy. This is not psychology. This is brain changing.

Comfort. Don't know about you, but I strive for comfort. Some people dress for fashion. I dress for comfort. When it comes to my home and office, comfort rules. Same goes for my mind. What I put in my head either satisfies a purpose, or I work at getting it out of my head. Things that make me anxious, sad, angry, unhappy, these are things that don't match a comfortable purpose. How do I get them out of my head? Usually, I transform them.

Transformation is very important to understand. The bad stuff that happens doesn't go away because we ignore it. However, we can change the bad stuff through transformation. How? When it comes to our thinking about bad stuff, we can mold those thoughts into something we can handle. We can handle our brain (neural) circuitry because it is has plasticity. Do you have too much clutter in your mind that doesn't work? Lay down new circuits, build new pathways. This is done by our own influence upon those thoughts that run up and down the circuitry of our brains. Say this to yourself: "I create my thoughts. I can control my thoughts."

If this is getting too scientific for you, you'll be thinking it's too hard. It isn't hard at all. We'll back up and redefine a few key words.

Brain: we've all got one. It's the mushy gray best-computer-ever-built inside your skull.

Circuitry: each time you have a thought, your brain fires up a pathway and runs the thought along that circuitry, with the result being an emotion or feeling. Thoughts first, then feelings. When you have a happy thought, your brain fires up a pathway, the happy thought runs along circuitry which culminates into emotions or feelings. When you have an angry thought, your brain fires up a pathway and the angry thought runs along circuitry carrying your anger, with results being emotions or feelings born out of angry thoughts. Pretend you can see inside your head. Pretend you can count your happy circuitry pathways. Pretend you can count your anger paths. How many happy circuits do you think you have? Do you think you have more anger circuits? Is your answer depressing? Don't sweat it. You can learn to transform your negative thoughts into more positive thoughts by changing your brain's circuitry; and your resulting emotions and feelings will match the more positive thoughts. One of the exercises included with this workbook will be keeping track of your negative thoughts.

Twenty-eight days. That's not a misprint. I'm talking 28. That's how long it takes to tow yourself out from the bad ruts in your brain and build better circuits. There is a catch. If you don't stick with your new circuit construction every day, you won't get the quality of results you want. Think of this construction as building new roads inside your head, one day at a time, for 28 days in succession. The succession part is very, very, very important, because that's how our brains work. I'm not simply picking out a number. Most research supports the 21 days to make changes theory. I believe 21 days is a good number. Neuroscience research suggests 28 days is a much better number.

Pencil exercise. You need a brand new pencil. Every morning when you first get up, for the duration of 28 days, you will begin your day putting a pencil crossways in your mouth. Hold it with your mouth, not your teeth. The idea is you are simply allowing it to rest in your mouth, you are not gripping it with your teeth. Keep it there five minutes. The pencil exercise makes your smile muscles work. Simultaneously, your facial nerves are sending that message directly to your brain! That's the point. You are going to begin your day, every day, with five minutes of smiling. Regardless how you feel when you first wake up, the exercise tricks your brain into beginning the day with a happy affect, and the exercise can influence your day to contain a lot more smiles.

These are not difficult things to understand. Changing is difficult, and you already know this: anything you do often, that's the thing you get really good at doing. If you have a habit of negative thinking, you are really good at doing that. You have become expert at negative thoughts. Thoughts beget feelings, and feelings beget actions (behavior). You have negative thoughts, then you will have negative feelings. If your feelings are negative, your actions and behavior are, too. You do this often, you are an expert at creating your own experience.

You are going to get plenty of repetition in this workbook. If you think, "I already read that, so I don't need to read it again," you just missed the point, and you are missing the boat, too! Read every word of every page, and do every step of your exercises!

Think of this as a 28 day journey toward more comforting positive life experiences.

* * *

WHAT DO YOU NEED?

1. A new pencil. If it is difficult to hold a standard pencil in your mouth, find the type used by children while they learn how to write. These are wider in circumference. My favorite is called "My First Ticonderoga."
2. Four single subject, 70 sheet, wide ruled spiral notebooks.
3. Two liquid gel pens, any color ink.
4. A timer. Sunbeam makes a 60 minute kitchen timer, available in the cooking section of most grocery stores or dollar stores, which sells for less than five dollars.
5. A committed contract with yourself. If you want to experience the effects of this program, you have to commit to working it, everyday, for 28 days. You must read the workbook, work the exercises, and be willing to implement what you are learning into your daily life. You are changing very basic aspects of yourself. You are transforming your thinking. The process is gradual and the results are cumulative. You are in control of the cumulative effects this program will have on your life.

* * *

DAY ONE

Begin your day with your pencil exercise. ***Remember each time you do this exercise, set your timer for five minutes.*** This exercise allows your facial muscles to send messages to your brain that you are happy. Your brain responds by flooding itself with happy hormones.

* * *

Retreat to a quiet place where you will not be interrupted, and that includes turning off all phones. I want you to slowly read this (which is why it is written from your point of view) <u>while</u> you are performing the breathing exercise. This is another five minute exercise. Set timer.

I am sitting in a comfortable chair. I am sitting so that my spine is stacked, my back is straight, and I am not slouching. My head is balanced comfortably, not leaning forward nor backward. I have one hand on my stomach and I am pulling oxygen deep down throughout my body. As I inhale, and then exhale, I can imagine I am breathing air into every cell in my body. I notice my chest expands minimally when I inhale, and my stomach expands generously, and I know that means I am breathing correctly. I feel relaxed. I feel peaceful. I am aware of my breathing. I am taking an in-breath. I am releasing an out-breath. I will continue listening to my in-breath and my out-breath, peacefully, until my timer rings.

After doing this exercise, I notice how peaceful and calm my body feels. I notice my mind has new focus. I feel present in this moment of my life. I am not stressing. I am not worrying. I am allowing the fresh oxygen from my five minute breathing exercise to nourish my body and my mind. I know I am fine. Right now. Right here.

* * *

DAY TWO

Begin today with your pencil exercise. Set your timer for five minutes and keep the pencil in your mouth until the timer rings.

Follow by setting your timer for another five minutes and continuing with your breathing exercise. You can always go back and read the exercise to help you get started.

* * *

You need a wide rule 70 sheet spiral notebook. You need a comfortable writing pen. I prefer liquid gel pens with a wide grip because they glide easy and they are comfortable in your hand for a long time. You need your timer.

Find a quite comfortable desk or table where you will not be interrupted or disturbed and no one will be looking over your shoulder. For this exercise, pretend your notebook is a favorite pet (or friend) from your childhood. Write the name of that pet (or friend) on the front of the notebook.

You are ready. Define "trauma" by looking it up in your dictionary. Review the meaning several times. Now, define that one traumatic or disturbing event in your life that has most defined you. Trauma occurs at any age. Turn the event into a story and begin writing about it, as if you were talking in real time to that childhood pet (or friend). Set your timer for 20 minutes. Write about your most accurate feelings and thinking around the event (as if telling the pet). Write about its influence upon your life. Open the gates and explore, explore, explore how this event affected you. You are taking all the mess and chaos and turning it into a story you can manage and describe to your childhood pet (or friend). Write without any care to your spelling or grammar. Just write. Don't hold back. You are writing to express whatever comes out of you regarding this event. You are writing toward healing the damage this event has caused you. Remember, your childhood pet (or friend) is with you, keeping you safe, listening, not judging, only hearing you and caring for you. By bringing this event out of your brain's hippocampus storage, and putting it on paper, you are placing it front and center in your brain's frontal lobe where you can touch it, organize it, explore it. The activity of doing this will help you gradually understand how this trauma has affected you, and what effect it has had on your life.

* * *

DAY THREE

Begin today with your pencil exercise. Set your timer for five minutes and keep the pencil in your mouth until the timer rings.

Follow by setting your timer for another five minutes and continuing with your breathing exercise. You can always go back and read the exercise.

* * *

This is the second day of your journal exercise, and it is a repeat of yesterday.

Set your timer for 20 minutes. Write, as if for the very first time, about your most accurate feelings and thinking about your trauma. Write about its influence upon your life. Open the gates wider. Define how this event affected you. You are taking all the mess and chaos and turning it into a story you can manage and describe. Write without any care to spelling or grammar. Just write. You are writing to heal the damage this event has caused you. Remember, bringing this event out of your brain's hippocampus storage and putting it on paper places it front and center in your frontal lobe where you can touch it, organize it, explore it. The activity of doing this will help you gradually understand, you are the one who controls and manages how this event affects you, and how you can handle it towards the healing of your own life.

* * *

❊ DAY FOUR ❊

Begin today with your pencil exercise. Set your timer for five minutes and keep the pencil in your mouth until the timer rings.

Follow by setting your timer for another five minutes and continuing with your breathing exercise. You can always go back and read the exercise.

* * *

This is the third day of your journal exercise. It repeats Day One and Two.

Set your timer for 20 minutes.

Today, write a story about that trauma.

When you are finished, review your story. Notice that this is history.

* * *

DAY FIVE

Begin today with your pencil exercise. Set your timer for five minutes and keep the pencil in your mouth until the timer rings.

Follow by setting your timer for another five minutes and continuing with your breathing exercise. You can always go back and read the exercise to help you get started.

* * *

This is the last day of journal exercise. It is a repeat of Day One, Two and Three.

Set your timer for 20 minutes.

Write about the trauma. Write whatever you want to say about it. When your timer rings, say, "The End."

* * *

You have a whole new perspective on this event which you have never had before. You structure it. You manage it. You control it. The event cannot be in control of you or your life, unless you let it. It no longer has the power to define you, unless you let it. You have defined it, you have shared all the scary stuff surrounding this event with your favorite childhood pet (or friend), and the event can now be allowed to evaporate into the nothingness where it belongs.

You can tear all the pages you wrote out of the notebook and shred them or burn them.

* * *

✤ DAY SIX ✤

Begin today with your pencil exercise. Set your timer for five minutes and keep the pencil in your mouth until the timer rings.

Follow by setting your timer for another five minutes and continuing with your breathing exercise. You can always go back and read the exercise.

*   *   *

Pick a poem. Perhaps you have a favorite. Perhaps you never read poetry. Today, you are going to read poetry. One of my all time favorite poems is Robert Frost's "*The Road Not Taken*." If you can't think of a poem to use in this exercise, I can almost promise, you will love *this* poem. To find it, put both the poet's name and the poem title into your internet search engine. Print it out and use it for this exercise. If you have trouble memorizing the poem, simply carry it with you and read it while you walk.

Today's exercise is more important than you can imagine, and this, or similar exercise throughout the rest of your life, is crucial to your healthy brain. What is it? Simple. Integration. People have known for a long time, art integrates the brain. Art brings the right brain and left brain into partnership where they work well together. Art includes so much more than painting and drawing. Art includes those creative skills we all have, whether music, illustration, song, building birdhouses, writing, reciting, acting, making jewelry, sculpting clay, and you get the idea, art is a basic integrator for our brain. When our brain integrates the right and left sides, we are happier, we are smarter, we make better choices, we find more purpose in our life. Is that enough to make you memorize a poem? Doesn't matter. Like I said earlier, if you can't or don't have time to memorize your chosen poem, find and print out a poem. Pick a classic. Pick a good one. Now, go for a walk (if that is possible). Otherwise, retreat to the most aesthetic place you can find right now, and read or recite your poem. Read it, or recite it, three times in a row. Three times! Savor the words. Savor the images. Experience the feeling of having a balanced brain, if only for a few minutes.

* * *

☆ DAY SEVEN ☆

Begin today with your pencil exercise. Set your timer for five minutes and keep the pencil in your mouth until the timer rings.

Follow by setting your timer for another five minutes and continuing with your breathing exercise. In-breaths. Out-breaths. While you breath, listen to your heart beating.

* * *

Capture and manage a worry! Keep your spiral notebook with you today. When you catch yourself worrying, write a brief summary identifying **what** exactly you worry about. After you write the worry down in your notebook, imagine you can now let it go. Every time that worry returns, before you find yourself obsessing about it, pretend you are catching it in your hand, then releasing it into the atmosphere. Say to yourself, "I will worry about this during my WORRY TIME this evening."

If you keep thinking about your worry item, repeat your breathing exercise. When the worry thought enters your mind, say to yourself, "I am breathing in, I am breathing out." Replace the worry thinking with thoughts of your in-breath and out-breath. Your mind can have only one thought in the present moment at a time. Replacing worry items with thoughts of your in-breath and out-breath is a healthy way to focus on the present moment instead of drifting into your history worrying about things that are already over, or have not yet happened. You cannot change the past by trying to go back there. You cannot create the future by obsessing about it. You can influence your mind's health and happiness by replacing those disruptive thoughts with healthy thinking.

These are not easy to do. You are changing the way your brain is used to working. Practice is how it's done. Practice putting more useful thoughts into your head.

This evening, your day will end with a planned structured WORRY TIME. Pick one of your spiral notebooks. Set your timer for 10 minutes. Write your worries from the day. When your timer rings, reset your timer for another 10 minutes. This time, pick a solution for each of the worries you wrote down. Write the solutions in your notebook. You have just ended your day as part of the SOLUTION to your worries. You cannot be part of your own worries if you learn to take active steps toward the solutions. Recall that oft heard saying, you are part of the problem, or you are part of the solution. Do this exercise, do it EVERY evening before you go to bed during the remainder of this 28 day program. You will learn how to be part of the solution in your own circumstance, which is a big step toward changing the way you think!

* * *

DAY EIGHT

Begin today with your pencil exercise. Set your timer for five minutes and keep the pencil in your mouth until the timer rings.

Follow by setting your timer for another five minutes and continuing with your breathing exercise. In-breath. Out-breath. Listen to your life sounds.

*   *   *

By now, you are certainly on to the secret of lifelong happiness. Happiness is not the big stuff. It is not the upscale new house. It is not the expensive import automobile. It is not the winning lottery ticket. Happiness is the little stuff, spread out frequently, throughout your lifetime. Believe it or not, that moment you arrive home from work and are greeted by the unconditional love of your favorite dog or cat, that is an event responsible for more lasting happiness in your life than you can or will ever get from the occasional big stuff. Bet you seldom think of the many people who do things for you almost every day, things you look forward to (but take for granted), like waking up to a fresh cup of coffee, getting your mail, having your newspaper at your doorstep, driving down highways that function, driving across bridges that are safe, listening to your favorite music. All of these little bits that fall across a day are pleasurable! They are tiny specks of happiness that too often go unnoticed in our day, but they don't go unnoticed inside our head. When things please us, our serotonin sprinkler washes over our brain, and we feel content. Unfortunately, much of the time, we don't consciously recognize the little stuff and think, "I am grateful!"

Today, you are going to begin noticing where you feel gratitude. To make sure you know when, where and why you are grateful, your assignment begins with defining two words: **GRATEFUL and GRATITUDE**. Look them both up in a dictionary. Read the definition. Read it again. Read it a third time. Grab one of your notebooks. Write the definition of GRATEFUL in your notebook three times. Then, write the definition of GRATITUDE in your notebook three times. Got it? Okay. So, what are you most grateful for? Write your answer in your notebook.

* * *

This evening, your day will wind down with a planned structured WORRY TIME. Pick one of your spiral notebooks. Set your timer for 10 minutes. Write your worries from the day. When your timer rings, reset your timer for another 10 minutes. This time, pick a solution for each of the worries you wrote down. Write the solutions in your notebook. You are now part of the SOLUTION to your worries.

* * *

Now, you will complete your day with today's exercise. When you close your eyes, recall what you wrote in your notebook after today's question: *What are you most grateful for?*

* * *

DAY NINE

Begin today with your pencil exercise. Set your timer for five minutes and keep the pencil in your mouth until the timer rings.

Follow by setting your timer for another five minutes and continuing with your breathing exercise. You can feel yourself healing your mind and your body.

* * *

Pull out the notebook you used yesterday. Read the definition of grateful. Read the definition of gratitude.

Get ready to write in your notebook.

List FIVE things for which you are very grateful today.

After you've listed all five, is one of your gratitudes a person?

For each person you listed, your next assignment is to buy a card. A simple expression of your appreciation for them is not too difficult, is it? Find a card that says something like, "Just wanted to tell you I appreciate you." Put a stamp on the envelope, address it and mail it, or give it to them in person. Wouldn't you love to receive a card like that?

* * *

This evening, your day winds down with the planned structured WORRY TIME. If you forget how this is done, review yesterday's directions.

Joan Leslie Woodruff

* * *

When you close your eyes, recall what you wrote in your notebook after today's question: **What are five things you are grateful for today?**

DAY TEN

Begin today with your pencil exercise. Set your timer for five minutes and keep the pencil in your mouth until the timer rings.

Follow by setting your timer for another five minutes and continuing with your breathing exercise. In-breath. Feel your happiness. Out-breath. Let your worries evaporate.

* * *

CBT and RET: Cognitive Behavioral Therapy and Rational Emotive Therapy. Both address our thoughts and feelings and spring from the position that our thinking creates our emotions, and our thoughts about ourselves result in positive or negative experiences in life. Science has backed these theories up for a long time. My experiential work as a therapist has backed up the accuracy of both theories, too. My personal experience a few years ago with serious depression solidified my already firm position: CBT and RET are effective methods leading to better, happier, more positive lives.

ANTS is an acronym for *automatic negative thoughts.* When you have a thought, the activity of simply having the thought registers in several ways which can be measured. Another activity which is measurable is what happens after the thought. Depending on the type of thought, your brain secretes chemicals. Your brain is bathing itself in good-feeling chemistry, or it is bathing itself in bad-feeling chemistry. Want to practice this? Let's practice. Set your timer for five minutes.

Close your eyes and imagine you are sitting beneath a beautiful shade tree in an equally beautiful countryside. It is a peaceful day. The weather is lovely. You are calm. You are without a care. You are relaxed. Life could not be better than this. Stay with this pleasurable experience until your timer rings. Open your eyes. Take two deep breaths.

Set your timer for two minutes. Close your eyes and imagine you are stuck in a traffic jam. The cars are not moving. You are glancing at your watch. You have a very important appointment in less than ten minutes. You are going to be late and you can't find your cell phone. You are worried you will not make the appointment at all. You are stuck in this traffic jam until your timer rings. Open your eyes. Take ten slow, deep breaths.

I purposefully let you have longer with your brain's feel-good chemistry. The purpose of the exercise is simple. When you have a good experience, your brain releases neurotransmitters. Specifically, it bathes itself in serotonin (hydroxytryptamine) and endorphins (hormones making active the body's opiate receptors). These are your natural highs.

I am sure two minutes stuck in traffic was long enough to notice cortisone (one of the glucocorticoids) building up. The resulting adrenaline rush isn't necessarily a good feeling.

What the exercise demonstrates is: your thoughts produce emotions, and your emotions result in the actions you take. Your behavior is an extension of your thoughts. Problem with this is obvious, don't you think? Do you believe your thoughts are all **TRUE?** Would you be surprised to know, universities have conducted studies for years regarding the accuracy of thoughts. The result? **Most of our thoughts are not true!**

How many thoughts do you imagine you have in one day? How many of those thoughts are negative? How often are you telling yourself negative things that aren't even true? An example might be: "I am not smart enough." Multiply that thought by hundreds of times. Recall now what we said a few days ago: What you do most often is what you are best at doing. If you tell yourself, "I am not smart enough," hundreds of times everyday, I imagine you have created a very ingrained circuit in your brain that agrees with you. Operative word here is *you.* YOU are the one who created that circuit in your brain. YOU are the one who can stop creating that circuit and put something more useful in its place. We will be actively doing just that during the next four days.

* * *

This evening, your day will wind down with a planned structured WORRY TIME.

Lights out, close your eyes, and before you fall asleep, ***think of five things you were grateful for today.***

* * *

❦ DAY ELEVEN ❦

Begin today with your pencil exercise. Set your timer for five minutes and keep the pencil in your mouth until the timer rings.

Follow by setting your timer for another five minutes and continuing your breathing exercise. While you breath, inhale happiness. Exhale negativity.

* * *

You learned on Day Ten that you spend most of your time in thought telling yourself fiction. Today you are going to make a list of the 15 most *negative* things you think about. I am providing you a *sample list.* Some of these items might be things you tell yourself about yourself. If they are, they will be part of your list. To arrive at your 15 common negative thoughts, carry your notebook with you today, and every time you catch yourself having a thought that is uncomfortable (negative) write it down.

Sample List of Negative Thoughts

1. Angry
2. Mean
3. Sad
4. Ugly
5. Stupid
6. Weak
7. Insecure

8. Alone
9. Unloved
10. Guilty
11. Scared
12. Failure
13. Fake
14. Incapable
15. Worthless

* * *

This evening, your day will wind down with a planned structured WORRY TIME. Lights out, close your eyes, and before you fall asleep, ***think of five things you were grateful for today.***

* * *

DAY TWELVE

Begin today with your pencil exercise. Set your timer for five minutes and keep the pencil in your mouth until the timer rings.

Follow by setting your timer for another five minutes and continuing with your breathing exercise. In-breaths make you wise. Out-breaths let go of troubles.

*   *   *

Today you are keeping track of your thoughts. Well, not all of your thoughts; you are keeping track of your list of negative thoughts. You need your notebook. Write your list of 15 negative thoughts. Every time you catch yourself having any of those thoughts, make a check or an *x* next to the thought. For instance, pretend the fifth thought on your list is *insecure.* Pretend, at the end of the day, you've caught yourself feeling insecure seven times. This is what your notebook entry would look like:

5. INSECURE *x x x x x x x*

This is not difficult to do, but it will take practice and commitment on your part. This is also one of the most important aspects of changing the way your brain sabotages you, or rather, changing the way you allow your brain to sabotage you.

Joan Leslie Woodruff

* * *

This evening, your day will wind down with a planned structured WORRY TIME. Lights out, close your eyes, and before you fall asleep, **think of five things you were grateful for today.**

* * *

DAY THIRTEEN

Begin today with your pencil exercise. Set your timer for five minutes and keep the pencil in your mouth until the timer rings.

Follow by setting your timer for another five minutes and continuing with your breathing exercise. While you breath, let your only thoughts be about your breathing.

* * *

Today you are continuing work with your list of 15 negative thoughts. Write down a column including all 15. Keep track, exactly like you did yesterday, by making marks next to each thought, each time you catch yourself having the thought. This time, at the end of the day, you are going to challenge your thoughts.

How do you challenge thoughts? Easy! Ask yourself, ***"Is it true?"***

Use your journal. Next to each thought, ask if it's true. Answer "yes" or "no."

* * *

This evening, your day will wind down with a planned structured WORRY TIME. Lights out, close your eyes, and before you fall asleep, ***think of five things you were grateful for today.***

* * *

DAY FOURTEEN

Begin today with your pencil exercise. Set your timer for five minutes and keep the pencil in your mouth until the timer rings.

Follow by setting your timer for another five minutes and continuing with your breathing exercise.

* * *

Today is a repeat of yesterday. You are continuing work with your list of 15 negative thoughts. Write down a column including all 15. Keep track, exactly like you've been doing, by making marks next to each thought, each time you catch yourself having the thought. At the end of the day, you are going to challenge your thoughts.

Use your journal. Next to each thought, ask ***"Is it true?"*** Answer "yes" or "no."

* * *

This evening, your day will wind down with a planned structured WORRY TIME. Lights out, close your eyes, and before you fall asleep, ***think of five things you were grateful for today.***

* * *

DAY FIFTEEN

Begin today with your pencil exercise. Set your timer for five minutes and keep the pencil in your mouth until the timer rings.

Follow by setting your timer for another five minutes and continuing with your breathing exercise.

* * *

Today's assignment is a repeat of yesterday. You are continuing work with your list of 15 negative thoughts. List a column including all 15. Keep track, exactly like you've been doing, by making marks next to each thought, each time you catch yourself having the thought. At the end of the day, you are going to challenge your thoughts.

Use your journal. Next to each thought, ask ***"Is it true?"*** Answer "yes" or "no."

* * *

This evening, your day will wind down with a planned structured WORRY TIME.

Lights out, close your eyes, and before you fall asleep, ***think of five things you were grateful for today.***

* * *

DAY SIXTEEN

Begin today with your pencil exercise. Set your timer for five minutes and keep the pencil in your mouth until the timer rings.

Follow by setting your timer for another five minutes and continuing with your breathing exercise.

* * *

Today you are going back through your journal. Review your list of negative thoughts. Review your challenges each day to each thought. You've been challenging each of your fifteen negative thoughts with the question: Is it true?

Today, continue keeping track of how often you have the same or similar negative thoughts. At the end of the day, your assignment is to challenge each thought with the question: **"How does that thought make me feel about myself?"**

Write down your answer (for each thought).

* * *

This evening, your day will wind down with a planned structured WORRY TIME. Remember, our greatest talent in life is upsetting ourselves. We are learning a healthier skill.

Lights out, close your eyes, and before you fall asleep, **think of five things you were grateful for today.**

* * *

DAY SEVENTEEN

Begin today with your pencil exercise. Set your timer for five minutes and keep the pencil in your mouth until the timer rings.

Follow by setting your timer for another five minutes and continuing with your breathing exercise. Breathing exercises are always available to us, regardless where we are. When we get obsessive thoughts in our head, replacing the thoughts with concentration on our breathing is often a good way to break the obsessive circle of thoughts.

* * *

Keep your notebook with you today. You are not working off your list of negative thoughts. You are writing down those negative thoughts you have most often. When you have a thought that causes you to feel uncomfortable (negative) jot it down in your notebook.

At the end of the day, process each negative thought that you've jotted down in the three ways demonstrated below. For example, if one of your persistent negative thoughts is, "I can't do this," I want you to process it as follows:

"I can't do this." Is that true? (Answer and write down your answer.)

"I can't do this." How does that thought make me feel? (Answer and write down your answer.)

"I can't do this." Would I be better off letting that thought go? (Answer and write down your answer.)

Continue this exercise for EVERY negative thought you had today (and wrote in your notebook). Answer all three questions for every negative thought. It is important that you write everything into your notebook. Catching those negative thoughts, and beginning the work of processing them this way, will go a long way to helping you change your life for the better.

* * *

This evening, your day will wind down with a planned structured WORRY TIME. Lights out, close your eyes, and before you fall asleep, ***think of five things you were grateful for today.***

* * *

DAY EIGHTEEN

Begin today with your pencil exercise. Set your timer for five minutes and keep the pencil in your mouth until the timer rings.

Follow by setting your timer for another five minutes and continuing with your breathing exercise. Listen to the quiet in your soul while you breath.

* * *

Keep your notebook close. You are to continue writing down those negative thoughts you have most often. At the end of the day, pick the three negative thoughts that you believe are the most destructive.

At the end of the day, process those three thoughts, using the same three questions.

First thought: Is that true? (Write down your answer.)

First thought: How does that thought make me feel? (Write down your answer.)

First thought: Would I be better off letting that thought go? (Write down your answer.)

Continue this exercise (all three questions) for the second and third negative thoughts. It is important that you write everything into your notebook. Remember, *catching those negative thoughts, and beginning the work of processing them this way, will go a long way to helping you change your life for the better.*

Joan Leslie Woodruff

* * *

This evening, your day will wind down with a planned structured WORRY TIME. Lights out, close your eyes, and before you fall asleep, **think of five things you were grateful for today.**

DAY NINETEEN

Begin today with your pencil exercise. Set your timer for five minutes and keep the pencil in your mouth until the timer rings.

Follow by setting your timer for another five minutes and continuing with your breathing exercise. You are learning to master perfect focus with this exercise. Focus increases IQ.

* * *

Consistent negative thoughts about others are not only destructive to how you feel about yourself, they are relationship enders. You cannot build onto your life if you are an island, which translates into: we all have (or need) relationships. Marriage and family are the first you probably think about, but you have relationships with all the people you regularly come across in your day. Your assignment today involves writing down the one most negative thought you have about the person you are closest to. You are going to work this as a process. Here is an example:

"He never appreciates me." Is that true? If you answer "yes" I want you to show proof that your belief is a fact. (Write down your answer.)

"He never appreciates me." How does that thought make me feel? (Write down your answer.)

"He never appreciates me." Would I be better off letting that thought go? (Write down your answer.)

Joan Leslie Woodruff

* * *

We've been highlighting how you use your thoughts. Remember this saying, "You are what you think?" I remember it well. When I was a child, and I'd launch into a rumor, or gossip, or other negative speech regarding one of my schoolmates, my mother would tell me, "You are what you think." She meant, if you think about the content of a rumor long enough, you will begin to believe it. Her position on rumors was they were hurtful and mean. The result of thinking about the content of rumors or gossip was that I'd filled my head with ugliness. I did not want to fill my head with ugliness. My mother was a wise person.

The consequences of that lesson helped me be a good friend to my friends, and compassionate toward others. I have not always been a good friend to myself, nor have I always been compassionate to others. When I fall into such a mindless rut, I don't feel happy. I'm not sure I even feel well! It is these times in my day when I most recognize ***I must challenge my thoughts***. It is also very important to recognize, not only must I challenge negative thoughts I have about myself, I absolutely must challenge negative thoughts I have about others, starting with those others who are closest to me. Creating fiction in our minds about other people is ridiculous; and, ***creating fiction in our minds about what we think other people think is a life crasher.***

Today you need one of your spiral notebooks. Write down three things you believe the person closest to you thinks about you. Example:

"He thinks I'm stupid."

"He thinks I'm ugly."

"He thinks I'm not interesting."

Now, I want you to challenge each of your responses by asking if it's true; and if you believe it's true, find supporting evidence. Note, if you do find supporting evidence (that this particular person thinks negative things about you), you might want to have a sit-down-serious conversation with that person. Surrounding ourselves with people who truly think negative things about us is like swimming with rocks in our pockets. Remember, the negative things another person thinks about you are as likely to be fiction as the negative things you think about them, or about yourself!

* * *

This evening, continue addressing the things you worried about with problem solving. By now, you may notice you are worrying about far less during the day than two weeks ago. You most likely are also doing active problem solving during real time when the worry first arises. This is becoming one of those things you will get better at the more you do it. It is a skill you can use for the rest of your life.

Now, pick one of your spiral notebooks. Your assignment this evening is to **write a letter to yourself.** Tell yourself what you are learning about yourself. Pay attention to the way you talk to yourself, and decide which parts of your letter empower you to do well, and which parts of your letter are part of your negative perception. Review your letter. Is it true?

Lights out, close your eyes, and before you fall asleep, **think of five things you were grateful for today.**

* * *

DAY TWENTY

Begin today with your pencil exercise. Set your timer for five minutes and keep the pencil in your mouth until the timer rings.

Follow by setting your timer for another five minutes and continuing with your breathing exercise. By now you recognize this is a very healthy exercise. Not only are you oxygenating your brain and body, you are allowing your mind adequate time to bring **YOU** into this moment, right here, right now, and that is something science tells us will **boost our focus and IQ**.

* * *

Today your assignment requires writing the following affirmation on an index card: *"I will be mindful of what I say to myself. I will practice <u>not</u> being critical of myself."*

This seems like such an easy exercise. It is probably not as easy as you think, but it is one of the most important SELF TALKS you can have with yourself.

Today, at the top of every hour, take the time to pull out your affirmation card and read it several times. If you can read it aloud, please do so. We tend to have more retention in seeing and hearing (which is why teachers like audiovisual).

* * *

During your evening, address a couple of things you worry about using your problem solving exercise. By this day, you have learned a few things about *worry.* Worry creates a mental image in our mind, and our brain responds to the image as if it is real. MOST of the time, that worry stuff *is not real.* Worry is a choice. You can choose to worry, or choose not to worry. If you are going to worry, set aside a worry time at the end of your day, and follow each worry with PROBLEM solving. Remember, worry is a thought, and thoughts are often not facts. Worry exhausts us.

Continue with last evening's letter exercise: ***write a letter to yourself.*** Tell yourself what you are learning about yourself. Pay attention to the way you talk to yourself, and decide which parts of your letter empower you to do well, and which parts of your letter are part of your negative perception. Review your letter. Is it true?

Lights out, close your eyes, and before you fall asleep, ***think of five things you were grateful for today.***

* * *

DAY TWENTY-ONE

If you are reading this, I'm assuming you made it to this point, have worked all your exercises, and have committed to changing your life for the better. Begin the day with your pencil exercise. Set your timer. While your smile muscles are sending happy messages to your brain, notice how different your day starts off because of this simple exercise. Remember what happens when you trick your face into smiling. Your facial nerves don't know they are being tricked. Your smile muscles are active, and the message going straight to your brain is that **YOU ARE HAPPY**. Even after your timer rings and you take the pencil out of your mouth, your brain thinks you are happy. <u>*GUESS WHAT? You ARE happy*</u>. By following this smiling exercise with another five minutes of IN-BREATH, OUT-BREATH breathing exercises, all the while keeping your thoughts on in-breaths and out-breaths, you are training your brain to focus. A brain with here and now focus is a brain without stress, without anxiety. That raises your IQ. In seven days, your workbook program ends; but, you will want to continue including these brain-healthy activities into your life often. Imagine, after one year, how different you will feel, and how much healthier your brain can be, by simply throwing in these two exercises most mornings!

Go ahead, set your timer, and concentrate on your breathing for five minutes.

* * *

You know this. I know this. When we hang on to our grudges, our resentments, we are blaming someone else for our thoughts, our feelings and our actions. We both know this, too: Forgiveness is for YOU. Forgiveness of others helps you take that first step toward healing and letting go of whatever it is you've been clutching close for too long. Resentment and grudges *do not hurt the person who is the target of your feelings.* Your inability to forgive them harms you!

Today you are replacing your resentment with a **Forgiveness Plant.** I am taking for granted you can afford a tiny plant, a small plant, a medium plant, or a full size young tree. Any type plant will work, as long as it requires some water and care at least once a week. This is a wonderful exercise, and you will want to remember it, and do this again anytime you are spending precious moments of your life resenting another person.

Sit with your new plant. Notice how it looks. Notice how it grows. Notice how it makes you feel. Especially, notice it will not survive if you don't attend to its care.

Today, every time you feel the flames of resentment arising in you toward another, STOP and pay attention to your plant. Take care of your plant. Talk to it. Listen to it. It is alive, and in its own way, it knows you are there, it knows it needs your help.

At the end of the day, you will have learned two very important truths. The first is, to maintain resentment, anger and grudges toward another, you spend time keeping those negative sentiments alive and well. ***You are watering that resentment and anger.*** You are feeding it. You are keeping it very much alive in your life. The second is, you could provide that energy toward nurturing something beautiful, keeping it alive and well. Your new plant is a lovely reminder, every time the flames of your resentment swell up inside you, you are the one having those thoughts. Dowse the flames, and transform your energy into nurturing your new plant, instead. In the end, you will have a lovely rooted friend who replaces that old angry fire. When that happens, you will be on your way to forgiving, because forgiveness is for you. Forgiveness does not condone harm another caused you; but, forgiveness is compassion in your soul to let it go.

*   *   *

This evening, your end-of-day assignments follow:

Write a letter to a person YOU harmed. Apologize. Ask their forgiveness. Be deeply, sincerely honest. When your letter is complete, you can throw away, or otherwise destroy, your letter. The activity of allowing this much truth out of the dark and into the light of day helps you forgive yourself for harming another. Truth is, we harm others, too. All the suffering in our lives was not caused by another or others. Much of our suffering is caused by our unkindness or lack of compassion for others, because there will always be a turnaround effect.

Lights out. Think of the three best people you have ever known. Think of why you are grateful for having known these people. Afterward, concentrate on your in-breath, and your out-breath, until you fall asleep.

* * *

DAY TWENTY-TWO

Set your timer for five minutes. Begin your day holding your pencil in your mouth. Never forget, happiness is contagious, even if you have to trick your brain into being happy!

Set your timer for five minutes. Concentrate on your in-breath and out-breath.

* * *

You have learned to be good at catching and noticing your negative thoughts. You have learned how to challenge negative thoughts, which helps take away their power over you. Your assignment today is to begin noticing, as you catch and challenge negative thoughts, that there are variations in their style. Sometimes it is simply the noting of the style of your negative thought that makes it possible to transform your thoughts into positive ones.

1. **All or Nothing.** This type of thinking leads us down the path of "always." In other words, all or nothing thinking sticks us into believing things like: "If I don't win today, I will always fail." "If I don't get a raise this time, I will never succeed." This is stuck-in-the mud thinking, and doesn't give us wiggle room to get out.
2. **Jumping to conclusions.** This thinking races us head-on into a brick wall. We are quick to believe things such as: "I'm gonna fail." "I can't do this." "They said 'no' last time I asked for a raise,

so they'll just say 'no' again." This type thinking predetermines our doom!
3. **Filtering.** This one is a sneaky quick method of self destruction. As negative thinkers, we can dismiss ten great things that happened in our week after we have ONE bad experience. We filter out ALL the good stuff, and only pay attention to the bad stuff.
4. **Mind readers.** We are great mind readers. Just by looking at another person, we can tell that they are thinking we are incompetent, we are ugly, we are stupid, we are failures. The real truth here is that we have no idea what other people are thinking, and when truth be revealed, most people are not thinking about us at all.
5. **Should.** Telling ourselves "I should have done this," or "I should have said that," is how we, as negative thinkers, punish ourselves constantly for not being perfect.
6. **Over generalizing (labels).** This is a form of slandering that we do to ourselves! Negative thinkers tend to accept unfair labels from others; and, as if we don't have enough of those, we tend to give ourselves labels.

* * *

After reading and reviewing these six common types of negative thinking, you are ready for today's assignment. You need a notebook. Catch and write down a minimum of 10 negative thoughts you have today. At the end of the day, decide which type of negative thought each one is, and write the type down next to the thought. By understanding more about your negative thought patterns, you can challenge them more easily.

* * *

This evening, your end-of-day assignments are:

Write a letter to a person who gave you negative labels. Be deeply, sincerely honest with yourself, and notice how often you have allowed this person's labels to stick on you. Tell that person they do not have power over you anymore. Tell them the labels are part of their own negative thoughts, and you refuse to own them. Tell them that by giving those labels to you, they were trying to unstick them from themselves. Tell them you understand that somewhere in their life, someone unfairly gave them those labels. Finish the letter, and throw it away. After you throw it away, you now recognize, the labels are not yours. You don't own them. You won't wear them anymore. They don't belong to you.

Lights out. Think of the three best things you have ever done for another/others. Think of why you are grateful for having done what you did. Afterward, concentrate on your in-breath, and your out-breath, until you fall asleep.

* * *

❦ DAY TWENTY-THREE ❦

Set your timer for five minutes. Begin your day holding your pencil in your mouth. Remember, happiness is contagious, even if you have to trick your brain into being happy!

Set your timer for five minutes. Concentrate on your in-breath and out-breath. You know this helps keep your brain healthy, and it helps raise your IQ.

* * *

Your assignment today is to make a list of 15 positive thoughts. Remember, positive thoughts are those that make you feel comfortable. Here are examples:

1. Comforted
2. Soothed
3. Safe
4. Relaxed
5. Energized
6. Special
7. Wonderful
8. Loved
9. Loving
10. Capable
11. Talented

12. Attractive
13. Accepted
14. Smart
15. Brilliant

* * *

Write your 15 positive items on an index card. Carry it with you today. Every time you have an uncomfortable thought, practice replacing that negative thought with one of the items from your positive list. Example:
"I am so dumb." . . . replace with "I am so smart."
"I am all alone." . . . replace with "I am loved."

* * *

End your day today by watching something humorous on television or the internet before you go to bed. I find the those priceless antique **"I Love Lucy"** shows are extremely helpful in adding light humor to the end of any day.

Lights out. Recall one person who is grateful for having YOU in their life. Recall one person you are grateful for having in YOUR life.

* * *

DAY TWENTY-FOUR

Set your timer for five minutes of smiling with your pencil in your mouth.

Set your timer for five minutes of breathing. Notice how calm you feel.

* * *

Today you need a spiral notebook. Keep it with you. Each time you have a negative thought, practice transforming the thought into positive thoughts. How? Simple. Replace the negative words with words from your positive word list. Do this consciously, all day! Write down as many negative thoughts as you catch and transform. Example: "No one likes me." Transformed: "I am a good person and my friends love me."

How are you feeling? Looking back, thinking of how you felt at the end of your days a month ago. If you've been working every day, every assignment, you have successfully begun upgrading your brain's circuitry for the better. When the brain is healthy, you feel good. When your thoughts are good, your brain is healthy. Simplistic? Yes, but it's also true.

Your wind-down-the-day assignment is also simple. Find a quiet peaceful place in your home where you can be undisturbed for 5 minutes. Set your timer. Close your eyes. Your life is like a summer lake. The sun is setting. The water is calm. The air is fresh and wonderful. You can hear a breeze lightly moving in and out of the leaves on the trees. You feel good. You feel special. You notice your breathing. In-breaths.

Joan Leslie Woodruff

Out-breaths. You are smiling. You continue listening to the gentle waves across the lake while you concentrate on your breathing.

Lights out. Think of two friends who you are very grateful to have known. Think of two friends who are very grateful for having known you.

DAY TWENTY-FIVE

Set your timer for five minutes of smiling with your pencil-in-mouth exercise.

Set your timer for five minutes of breathing. Your breathing refreshes you.

* * *

YOU FEEL WHAT YOU THINK!

You should know this by now. The thoughts in your mind will either make your life better, or they will wreak havoc on your every attempt to have a good life. Isn't it worth your time, your efforts, your commitment to practice paying more attention to how you think?

Your assignment today requires a spiral notebook. Catch and record at least two of your most troublesome thoughts, those things you keep thinking that are interfering with having a better day.

List each negative thought. Under each thought provide five alternative positive thoughts.

Practice, for the remainder of the day, replacing those negative thoughts with positive thoughts from your list.

* * *

This evening's wind down exercise begins with a set of affirmations:

1. I can choose my thoughts.
2. I know good thoughts make good days.

3. I am worthwhile.
4. I can do this. I can change my life by changing my thoughts.

* * *

Lights out. Notice your lungs pulling oxygen in through your nose. Noticing your lungs pushing air out from your mouth. Notice your two feet while you notice your breathing. Notice your two knees while you notice your breathing. Notice your two hips while you notice your breathing. Notice your spine while you notice your breathing. Notice your two hands while you notice your breathing. Notice your two wrists while you notice your breathing. Notice your two elbows while you notice your breathing. Notice your two shoulders while you notice your breathing. Notice your ribs while you notice your breathing. Notice your two ears while you notice your breathing. Notice your nose. Notice your mouth. Notice your two eyes. Notice you are focused on your in-breaths, and your out-breaths. Notice how peaceful you feel.

* * *

DAY TWENTY-SIX

Set your timer for five minutes of smiling with your pencil-in-mouth exercise.

Set your timer for five minutes of breathing. In-breaths. Out-breaths. You feel good.

* * *

Let's put a toolbox together with skills to help you through future rough spots. You know life isn't always easy. You know it is not realistic to expect to always be happy. You know good things happen. You know bad things happen. You understand we control our thoughts, but we do not control others, and we do not control the world. You also know, ***you can arm yourself to get through those times that put our strength to the test.***

1. When bad feelings take over, ask yourself, "What was going through my mind just before I had bad feelings? What am I telling myself? Is it true?"
2. Negative thoughts are like garbage. You can transform them. You can turn the garbage into flowers by replacing bad thoughts with positive thoughts. You can do this.

Pick a negative thought you are having. What is in your mind right now? Is this true?

Imagine that thought is a pile of garbage. Imagine you plant a flower on top of the garbage, and the flower takes over. Imagine the bad thought is replaced by the flower.

Of course you can do this; but, **<u>you</u>** have to do it. You cannot hire someone to do this for you. You cannot take a pill to do this for you. You cannot wake up and suddenly be able to do this. You must practice, practice, practice.

Remember, you get very, very good at doing that which you do frequently. ***If you learn to frequently replace the garbage with flowers, you will get very good at having a happier life***.

* * *

Finish your day by going back through your workbooks, find the end-of-day exercise that works best for you.

Lights out. Do the exercise that works best for you.

* * *

DAY TWENTY-SEVEN

Set your timer for five minutes of smiling with your pencil-in-mouth exercise.

Set your timer for five minutes of breathing. You can feel your IQ has increased!

* * *

Today, review your workbooks. Find the exercise you most enjoyed.

Your assignment today is, do that exercise.

* * *

Lights out. Do the end-of-day exercise you most enjoy.

* * *

❖ DAY TWENTY-EIGHT ❖

GUESS WHAT? You are almost finished with your workbook!
Set your timer for five minutes of smiling exercise with your pencil in mouth.

Set your timer for five minutes of breathing. Focus only on your in-breath and out-breath.

* * *

Neuroscience has shown repeatedly, our brain has enormous neuroplasticity. We can change our brain by changing what we put into our brain. We can be more selective with our thoughts because we now understand, our thoughts create our feelings, and our feelings lead to our actions and behavior.

What about all those days ahead when you can't quite get up to speed? You know those days are going to befall us. Life promises, regardless how hard we work at anything, bad stuff will happen when we least expect it. I know, I've had some really bad sad stuff in my life. I also know, working at those skills I possess which will get me through the worst of times, I do emerge a bit better off in thought and attitude. Using the tool box filled with your new skills, you can do wonders.

Considering the skills you learned, here are some ***quick tricks to help you lift yourself*** out of a low spell:

1. Don't forget the pencil exercise. You are working smile muscles. The brief bath of neurotransmitters flooding over your brain will surely lift your mood.

2. When you suddenly feel unhappy, ask yourself, "What was I thinking right before I felt this way?" Remember, your thoughts are responsible for your feelings. Catch them and challenge them when they aren't working for you.
3. Too many negative thoughts can wreck your day. If you are having a really bad day, find your spiral notebook and write down the thoughts you are having. Begin processing them with the same three questions you learned earlier. Replace negative with positive words.
4. Breathing. This is a tool you always have with you. When you need a lift, set some time aside to breath. Don't do anything else. Just breath. Listen to your in-breath. Listen to your out-breath. Think only about breathing. Do this for a minimum of five minutes. The oxygen nourishes you, and the focus nourishes your brain.

* * *

Of course, **this workbook is not intended as a one-size-fits-all manual**. The audience who will most benefit from this includes people who believe they could feel more positive about their life, but don't quite know how. If your problems persist, and you are simply unable to pull yourself up from the low tides, you need more intensive help. See your personal physician, and do ask for a thorough physical exam. If all checks out physically, you might consider finding a therapist or psychologist to work with you one-to-one.

I hope you benefitted from this workbook, and I especially hope you don't stop practicing the new skills you learned. You might want to save this workbook and redo it once a year for several years in a row.

Remember, what you do often is what you get really good at doing. Get really good at this stuff. By the way, if you are hooked on what you can learn and do to make a difference in your own life, read my Reference List (following page), find work by any of the brilliant people listed, and go for the total overhaul! Keep life's mind games working for you.

Happy Trails!

PIONEERS WHO BLAZED THE BRAIN CHANGE TRAIL

Daniel Amen, MD. One of the "Change Your Brain" pioneers (and book author).

Aaron Beck, MD. Recognized founder of CBT (author of multiple related books).

James Gordon, MD. Author of depression recovery book, UNSTUCK.

Thich Nhat Hahn. Buddhist Monk. Teacher of peace. Teacher of mindfulness and meditation.

Jon Kabat-Zinn, PhD. Developed in-hospital programs for stress reduction and mindfulness.

Byron Katie. Developed "The Work," a highly useful technique, used to effectively change thoughts and behavior.

James W. Pennebaker, PhD. Developed therapeutic "Writing to Heal" program, and other highly effective writing techniques to improve mental health.

Dan Siegel, MD. Author of THE MINDFUL BRAIN, which examines thought affect on brain.

Socrates. Born in Athens, Greece around 460 BC. His Socratic Method relies on logic (truth).

❦ MY OTHER BOOKS ❦

Your Book. Exercise programs to accompany doctor and therapist treatments. Published in 1984 by Carl Chen, MD, and Joan Leslie Woodruff, MA OTR, Hand Surgery Practice and Rehabilitation Clinic, Fullerton, California.

Traditional Stories & Foods: An American Indian Remembers. Published in 1990 by Esoterica Press, Barstow, California. ISBN-13 9780943557021. ISBN-10 094355702X.

Neighbors. First edition published in 1993 by Third Woman Press, University of California, Berkeley, California. Reprinted for POD in 2007. ISBN-13 9780943219080. ISBN-10 0943219086.

The Shiloh Renewal. First edition published in 1998 by Black Heron Press, Seattle, Washington. ISBN-13 9780930773502. ISBN-10 0930773500.

Ghost in the Rainbow. Published in 2002 by Hats Off Books, Tucson, Arizona. ISBN-13 9781587361470. ISBN-10 1587361477.

Wishes & Windmills. Published in 2003 by Hats Off Books, Tucson, Arizona. ISBN-13 9781587362484. ISBN-10 1587362481.

The Shiloh Renewal. Published for audio cassette, compact disc, audio downloads, and audio CD in 2007 for distribution by

Joan Leslie Woodruff

Blackstone Audio Inc, and narrated by Rebecca Rogers. ISBN-13 9781433205897. ISBN-10 1433205912. (Six versions of audio available.)

Polar Bears in the Kitchen. Published in 2009 by Wheatmark Publishers, Tucson, Arizona. ISBN-13 9781604942934. ISBN-10 1604942932.

www.ingramcontent.com/pod-product-compliance
Lightning Source LLC
Chambersburg PA
CBHW021007180526
45163CB00005B/1928